Acid Reflux

A Comprehensive Guide To Balancing Your Diet,
Reducing Heartburn And Reflux Symptoms

(Delicious Recipes To Naturally Relieve Heartburn And Prevent Acid Reflux From Worsening)

Pâmela-Lorne Langevin

TABLE OF CONTENT

Introduction 1

Chapter 1: What Exactly Is Acid Reflux?....................... 2

Chapter 2: The Acid Reflux Diet.....................................11

Chapter 3: Foods That May Be Included In Your Diet 28

Chapter 4: How Do Asd Blosker Work To Treat Acid Reflux? 32

Cashew Snaps 36

Broccoli And Sharp Cheddar Cheese Bte....................38

Chapter 5: A List Of Foods To Simply Avoid 40

Chapter 6: Diet Guide What Is Bland Diet?................50

Chapter 7: Best Herbs For Acid Reflux.......................54

Chapter 8: What Are The Stipulations Of Gatrorare? 62

Chapter 9: Control Your Symptoms Using The Acid Reflux Diet..72

Chapter 10: Is The Acid Reflux Diet A Good Option For You?...................79

Teriyaki Shrimp Sushi Bowl..85

Simple Chisken & Veggie Soup 89

Garlic-Infused Mashed Potatoes.....................................91

Introduction

When acid from the stomach flows back up into the esophagus, acid reflux occurs. This is a common occurrence, but it may result in complications or distressing symptoms, such as heartburn.

The lower esophageal sphincter (LES) may be weakened or injured, contributing to this condition. The LES normally closes to prevent stomach contents from entering the esophagus.

Dietary habits influence the amount of stomach acid produced. Eating the right foods is essential for controlling acid reflux or gastro esophageal reflux disease (GERD), a severe, chronic form of acid reflux.

Chapter 1: What Exactly Is Acid Reflux?

Acid reflux occurs when corrosive material from the stomach flows back up into the throat. Heartburn is the desire to consume that an individual with heartburn has. Recurrent acid reflux may indicate that a person has GERD.

Although people may use the terms interchangeably, indigestion, also known as acid reflux, is a side effect of heartburn, also known as gastroesophageal reflux (GER). Acid reflux has no relation to the heart, despite its name.

Gastroesophageal reflux disease (GERD) is a more severe form of gastroesophageal reflux (GER). Specialists will diagnose GERD when a patient's indigestion becomes a recurring complaint, typically more than twice per day for an extended period of time. GERD is most prevalent in Western nations, affecting an estimated 20% of the population.

Approximately 20% of Americans have GERD, and it is the most studied gastrointestinal disorder in the short-term setting. Approximately 60% of individuals with GERD are female. African Americans comprise the second-largest population of GERD sufferers, after white individuals.

Why do acid reflux episodes occur?

The stomach contains hydrochloric corrosive, a major strength that separates food and protects against microorganisms such as microorganisms.

The coating of the stomach is specially adapted to protect it from strong acids, but the throat is not protected. The gastroesophageal sphincter is a muscle ring that acts as a valve that allows food to enter the stomach but prevents it from backing up into the throat.

When this valve fails, stomach contents are once again expelled into the throat. This is acid reflux. As the corrosive ascends, the victim will experience a burning sensation in the throat. This is acid reflux.

These are additional frequent risk factors for acid reflux infection:

Eating massive dinners or sleeping immediately after a feast

Being overweight or large

Eating a heavy meal while lying on one's back or twisting at the midsection

Eating close to bedtime

Consuming specific food types, such as citrus, tomato, chocolate, mint, garlic, onions, or fiery or fatty food sources, can cause gastrointestinal distress.

Consuming specific beverages, such as liquor, carbonated drinks, espresso, or tea

Smoking

Taking medications for headaches, ibuprofen, certain muscle relaxants, or circulatory strain while pregnant.

How Acid Reflux Can Negatively Really impact Your Life

Acid reflux is a common condition that affects a large number of individuals. After a substantial meal, acid neutralizers are really helpful in mild cases. For certain individuals, heartburn is persistent and severe, and standard over-the-counter medications do not provide much relief in this regard. This is how indigestion can negatively really impact your life, and this is how you can reduce the side effects of heartburn.

Timing of meals

Intense indigestion or gastroesophageal reflux disease (GERD) can make meals agonizing. It may be difficult to consume anything without experiencing chest pain, nausea, and same difficulty swallowing. Traveling to restaurants can be hazardous due to the prevalence of heartburn triggers in nearly all foods. The vast majority of people with severe heartburn must easy cook at home with restricted flavors.

Sleep

It can be nearly impossible to sleep flat with acid reflux. Acidic and stomach contents can crawl up the throat, causing severe choking pain. Individuals with severe GERD may sleep poorly and awaken frequently during the night.

WORK

When afflicted, it can be difficult to concentrate on work, but certain work activities can alleviate heartburn symptoms. Specifically, bowing and lifting can cause a corrosive stream to rise into the throat. You may be able to obtain a note from your physician allowing you to simply avoid bowing and lifting, or you may be able to alter how you perform easy task to simply avoid side-effect eruptions. In spite of the fact that alterations can sometimes be easy made to provide relief at work, managing heartburn at work can be difficult and discouraging.

Extreme Agony

Sometimes, the chest pain associated with reflux can mimic the worsening of respiratory failure. It is common for people with indigestion to visit the emergency room during a severe attack, believing that something is seriously wrong or that their heart is causing the discomfort. Due to the fact that the nerve that runs along the throat and to the stomach is responsible for the autonomic sensory system, the side effects can be perplexing. Certain individuals with reflux may experience exceptional "coronary failure" pain in their left arm or heart palpitations. Typically, trauma centers can offer temporary relief with a "GI mixed drink" that resembles an acid neutralizer and desensitizing medication. They can guarantee that it is not your heart, but you will be encouraged to return to a specialist for testing to determine the severity of your acid reflux.

Chapter 2: The Acid Reflux Diet

Virtually every study on gastroesophageal reflux disease and acid reflux disease (ARD) identifies a poor diet as a contributing factor. In addition, it is simple to overindulge in sugary foods while neglecting mindful eating habits. While everyone's gut is unique and we all react to different foods in our own way, there are certain foods that appear to trigger acid reflux in certain individuals. Focus on removing these "repeat offenders" from your list as soon as possible. For good digestive health and relief from bloating, it is essential to consume organic, non-GMO foods as frequently as possible. Increasing fiber consumption, supporting healthy bacteria with foods rich in antioxidants and curcumin, easily reducing grain consumption, and consuming high-quality protein will also aid in restoring digestive health. In addition, incorporating these simple changes into your diet reduces risk factors such as inflammation, obesity, and the complications associated with severe forms of schizophrenia.

Here are some foods that can aid acid reflux and treat GERD:

• Kefir and yogurt aid in digestion and soothe the digestive tract by balancing healthy bacteria in the stomach. Choose fermented rrodust with live and active cultures and a 28 -hour fermentation time.

• Bone broth easy made from grass-fed beef, cooked slowly to extract vital compounds including collagen, glutamine, proline, and glusne.

• Fermented vegetables insluding kimshi and sauerkraut.

- Kombusha was entrusted with healthu bastera and rrobots.

- Apple cider vinegar assists in balancing stomach acid and alleviating the symptoms of acid reflux. Mix one teaspoon of raw apple cider vinegar with one cup of water and drink it five minutes before eating.

- Coconut water is rich in potassium and elestrolute, which assist in keeping the body hydrated. To help prevent acid reflux at night, drink water throughout the day and a glass before bed. Additionally, coconut water can be fermented into kefir, which adds additional probiotics to the stomach that individuals with acid reflux desperately need.

- Coconut oil is an excellent source of healthy fat that also has anti-inflammatory properties. A tableroon of sosonut ol dalu is to be consumed by Tru. rread it on rrouted grain bread or incorporate it into other foods, for instance. The lauric acid and other natural substances aid in combating inflammation, boosting the immune system, and eliminating parasites.

• Leafy green vegetables • Artichokes • Asparagus • Cucumber • Pumpkin and other uah • Wild-caught tuna and salmon

• Healthy fats that include soynut oil and ghee

• Raw sow's milk cheese • Almonds

Numerous of these foodstuffs are included n The GAPS diet, which focuses on whole foods and which I recommend to people with digestive problems. In addition to acid reflux, the GAPS diet can aid in the treatment of irritable bowel syndrome, intestinal permeability, attention deficit hyperactivity disorder, and numerous other conditions. In actuality, the GAPS diet consists primarily of fresh organic vegetables, grass-fed beef, and free-range chicken, as well as bone broth. It also contains digestive-soothing herbs such as aloe vera, red raspberry leaf, ginger, and fennel.

Stomach acid hitting the esophagus and causing discomfort and pain can cause reflux symptoms. If you have excess acid, you can incorporate the easily following foods into your diet to reduce acid reflux symptoms.

Your decision to try these specific foods to alleviate your symptoms should be based on your individual experiences with them, as none of these foods will cure your disease.

Vegetables

Naturally, vegetables are low in fat and sugar. Green beans, broccoli, asparagus, cauliflower, leafy greens, potatoes, and cucumbers are excellent options.

Ginger

Ginger has anti-inflammatory properties and is used as a natural treatment for heartburn and other gastrointestinal conditions. You can relieve symptoms by adding grated or sliced ginger root to meals or smoothies, or by drinking ginger tea.

Oatmeal

Oatmeal, a popular breakfast food, is a whole grain and a rich source of fiber. A high-fiber diet has been associated with a reduced risk of acid reflux. Rice and bread easy made with whole grains are additional sources of fiber.

Non-citrus fruits

Melons, bananas, apples, and pears, which are not citrus fruits, are less likely to cause reflux symptoms than acidic fruits.

lean meats and fish

Low-fat meats, such as chicken, turkey, fish, and seafood, can alleviate acid reflux symptoms. Try grilling, broiling, roasting, or poaching them.

The whites of eggs

Egg whites are a suitable substitute. However, egg yolks are high in fat and may exacerbate reflux symptoms.

Healthy lipids

Avocados, walnuts, flaxseed, olive oil, sesame oil, and sunflower oil are sources of healthy fats. Replace saturated and Trans fats with these healthy unsaturated fats and reduce your intake of saturated and Trans fats.

It is my responsibility to inform you that I am not prescribing any of these medications before we begin. This section is meant to inform you about some of the medications used to treat acid reflux. Are these medications healthy? Do they treat your acid reflux? You will understand as you continue reading. But for now, let's get to know them and assess their capabilities.

Many of these medications are available over-the-counter, so you do not need a prescription to obtain them; however, if you experience these symptoms for an extended period of time, it is important to see a doctor. Therefore, let's examine the various medications prescribed for acid reflux disease.

ANTACIDS

Antacids are, in my opinion, the most prevalent treatment for acid reflux diseases. As the name suggests, anti-acids contain basic chemicals that neutralize the acid in your stomach, preventing acid from refluxing into your esophagus and causing heartburn. The issue with antacids is that their effect is only temporary. They are typically expelled from the stomach in less than an hour, and the acid then re-accumulates, bringing you back to square one.

Therefore, the optimal time to take antacids is approximately one hour after meals, just before the onset of reflux symptoms. Since food slows the stomach's emptying, an antacid taken after a meal remains in the stomach longer and is therefore more effective.

Antacids are typically composed of aluminum, magnesium, or calcium.

Antacids containing aluminum have a tendency to cause constipation, whereas antacids containing magnesium have a tendency to cause diarrhea. Antacids containing both magnesium and aluminum are less problematic. (This is to demonstrate that drug dependence is a poor choice)

H2 BLOCKERS

After antacids, the H2 blockers are the next class of drugs used to treat acid reflux disease. There are H2 receptors within the cells of the stomach wall. Histamine's stimulation of these receptors results in acid secretion. Therefore, drugs were developed to block these receptors in order to reduce stomach acidity.

This category contains the medications cimetidine, ranitidine, nizatidine, and famotidine. All four are available without a prescription as over-the-counter (OTC) products. However, over-the-counter dosages are lower than prescription dosages.

H2 antagonists are most effective when taken 6 0 minutes before a meal, as histamine plays a crucial role in the stimulation of stomach acid. This is done so that the H2 blockers will be at their highest levels in the body easily following a meal, when the stomach is actively producing acid. H2 blockers can also be taken at bedtime to suppress acid production during the night.

PROTON PUMP INHIBITORS (PPI)

Proton pump inhibitors, in particular omeprazole, are the third type of drug designed specifically for acid-related diseases. When you take PPIs, they prevent the stomach from producing acid.

The advantage of a PPI over an H2 blocker is that the PPI completely and for a longer period of time inhibits acid production. In addition to treating the symptom of heartburn, PPIs protect the esophagus from acid, allowing the esophageal inflammation to heal.

PPIs are used when H2 blockers fail to adequately relieve symptoms or when complications of GERD develop.

Available PPIs for the treatment of GERD include lansoprazole, rabeprazole, pantoprazole, and esomeprazole in addition to omeprazole (gastroesophageal reflux disease).

PPIs should be taken one hour before meals. This is because PPIs are most effective when the stomach is actively producing acid, which occurs after meals. If the PPI is taken before the meal, it will be at its peak concentration in the body (after the meal) when the acid is being produced and will perform admirably.

PROMILITY DRUGS

Pro-motility drugs function by stimulating the esophagus and stomach muscles of the gastrointestinal tract.

Metoclopramide is an example of a drug approved for the treatment of GERD that promotes fertility. The contractions of the esophagus are strengthened and the pressure in the lower esophageal sphincter is increased by fertility drugs. Both effects are expected to reduce acid reflux. Nevertheless, these effects on the sphincter and esophagus are negligible. Therefore, it is believed that the primary effect of metoclopramide may be to accelerate stomach emptying, which would also be expected to reduce acid reflux. Pro-motility medications are most effective when taken 6 0 minutes prior to meals and again before bed.

FOAM BARRIERS

Foam barriers are a second class of medications used to treat acid reflux.

Foam barriers are an innovative treatment for GERD. Composed of an antacid and a foaming agent, these are either tablets OR liquids. As the tablet disintegrates and reaches the stomach, it transforms into a foam that floats on top of the stomach's liquid contents.

The foam forms a physical barrier against liquid reflux. In addition, the antacid attached to the foam neutralizes acid that comes into contact with it.

The best times to take the tablets are after meals (when the stomach is distended) and when lying down, as this is when reflux is most likely to occur. The only foam barrier consists of aluminum hydroxide gel, magnesium trisilicate, and alginate.

Typically, each of the medications listed above is effective in treating the symptoms and complications of GERD. However, occasionally they are not. The amount or number of drugs required for effective treatment is excessively high, making drug treatment unreasonable.

In such cases, acid reflux can also be effectively treated with surgery. Fundoplication or anti-reflux surgery is the medical term for the surgical procedure that is performed to prevent reflux.

FUNDOPLICATION (ANTI-REFLUX SURGERY) (ANTI-REFLUX SURGERY)

Throughout the fundoplication procedure, the fundus of the stomach is gathered, wrapped, and sutured around the lower end of the esophagus and the lower esophageal sphincter.

Chapter 3: Foods That May Be Included In Your Diet

If you wish to alleviate the symptoms of gastroesophageal reflux disease (GERD), you will likely have to eliminate certain foods from your diet. In this situation, it may be beneficial to be aware of alternative foods that are less likely to cause allergic reactions.

The easily following alternatives may prevent you from experiencing symptoms:

Items containing milk: Try milk, yogurt, cheese, and ice cream with reduced, low, or no fat instead of whole milk and full-fat dairy products.

You could also experiment with non-dairy alternatives to dairy products, such as almond or soy milk and non-dairy ice cream.

Replace high-fat baked goods such as biscuits, croissants, doughnuts, and sweet rolls with lower-fat options such as plain bread or rolls, pancakes, waffles, bagels, and low-fat muffins.

Meats and other sources of protein: Instead of fatty cuts of meat, fried meat, lunch meat, or sausages, try leaner cuts of meat, poultry without the skin, fish, tofu, or eggs.

Simply avoid citrus fruits such as oranges, lemons, limes, and grapefruit and consume any other safe fresh, frozen, or canned fruit or fruit juice.

Test out a variety of oil-free fresh, frozen, and canned vegetables: These vegetables can be substituted for fried or creamed vegetables, onions, tomatoes and tomato derivatives, and vegetable juices.

Soups Instead of creamy or tomato-based soups, choose broth-based or homeeasy made soups easy made with lean ingredients, such as low-fat or fat-free milk in place of cream.

Potatoes and other starchy foods: Instead of potato chips, french fries, risotto, or pasta with creamy or tomato-based sauces, try baked, boiled, or mashed potatoes, plain pasta or rice, or pasta with a low-fat milk-based sauce. You can also reduce the amount of fat and calories in your diet by avoiding potato chips, risotto, and pasta with tomato-based sauces.

Snacks Try crackers, pretzels, corn tortillas, low-fat hummus, and sliced fruits (other than citrus) or vegetables instead of fried chips, almonds, guacamole, cheese dip, or sour cream-based dips. Each of these alternatives is better for you.

Try substituting chocolate, cookies, cakes, and pastries with marshmallows, non-mint hard candies, angel food cake, gelatin desserts, fruit-based desserts, sherbet, or low-fat pudding when it comes to sweets and desserts.

Chapter 4: How Do Asd Blosker Work To Treat Acid Reflux?

Products similar to Pepcid AC are salled histamine H2 blockers, or acid bloskers. The production of tomash asd is diminished by acid blosker. Theu alleviate heartburn, indigestion, and upset stomach. Always follow the instructions on the label or consult with your healthcare provider regarding how to take the medication. Asd blockers you can purchase without a prescription include:

Persid Tagamet

Take your antidepressant regularly for as long as your doctor recommends, even if your symptoms improve or you no longer have any symptoms.

Stronger asid bloskers are rressrirtion medisations. These can be used to treat

GERD, stomach and duodenal ulcers, erosive esophagitis, and acid reflux. They function by decreasing the production of stomach acid. Your healthcare provider will provide a risk assessment for this type of acid reflux.

The United States of America Food and Drug Administration (FDA) reported elevated levels of a potential sarsenogen, NDMA, in ranitidine (Zantac) and nizatidine (Axed). If you are currently taking one of these medications, you should consult your doctor.

Exist any 'de effest' forms of ADHD blockers?

Side effects of asid bloskers inslude:

Headache.

Dizziness.

Diarrhea.

Inform your healthcare provider immediately if you experience any of the easily following serious side effects after taking an adrenergic blocker:

Confusion.

Quickly, please!

Bleeding.

painful throat.

Fever.

Abnormal heartbeat

Weakness or uncommon fatigue

Should I use both antacids and acid blosker to treat heartburn?

Your doctor may advise you to take antihistamines when you begin taking an antihistamine. Your symptoms will be controlled by antacids until the acid blockers take effect. If your doctor prescribes an antihistamine, take it one hour before (or one hour after) taking an antihistamine tablet.

Cashew Snaps

Ingredients

½ teaspoon baking soda

1/7 teaspoon salt

3 cups all-purpose flour

1 cup butter

3 cups packed brown sugar

2 fresh egg

1 cup chopped cashews

Directions

1. Preheat oven to 450 degrees F (2 710 degrees C). Lightly grease cookie sheet.
2. In a large bowl, cream together the butter, brown sugar, and egg.
3. Stir in the chopped cashews, baking soda, salt, and flour.
4. Drop by half teaspoon two inches apart onto greased cookie sheet.
5. Bake at 450 degrees F (250) for 25 to 30 minutes.

Broccoli And Sharp Cheddar Cheese Bte

Ingredients

- 1/2 tsp dried oregano
- 1/7 tsp salt
- 10 large eggs
- 2 cup broccoli, chopped very small
- 1/2 cup & 12 tsp cheddar cheese, shredded

Directions

1. Preheat the oven to 450 degrees Fahrenheit.
2. Spray a muffin tin with nonstick easy easy cook ing spray, or add a bit of easily melted coconut oil to each muffin cup and spread around.
3. In a large bowl whisk all of the eggs, until well blended, then add in the

cup of broccoli, oregano, salt and 2 /6 cup of cheddar cheese.
4. Mix well.
5. Pour the mixture into the each of the muffin cup distributing evenly.
6. Be careful not to overfill as it can overflow in your oven! I would also maybe recommend easily putting a baking sheet underneath your muffin tin, if you are worried about it.
7. Bake for 70 to 80 minutes, or until a toothpick comes out clean.
8. Easily Remove from the oven, and let cool for about 5-10 minutes, then take a knife around the side of each muffin and then scoop them out.
9. Can be kept in the fridge for up to 10 days.
10. Takes about 80 to 90 seconds to reheat in the microwave!

Chapter 5: A List Of Foods To Simply Avoid

Certain foods have been shown to cause problems for a large number of people, despite the fact that experts are divided as to whether or not foods actually cause reflux symptoms.

To begin managing your symptoms, you may wish to eliminate the easily following foods from your diet:

Fried and fatty foods may relax the lower esophageal sphincter (LES), allowing stomach acid to reflux more easily into the esophagus. Moreover, these foods prevent the stomach from emptying.

Eating high-fat foods increases the likelihood of developing reflux symptoms; therefore, easily reducing your daily fat consumption can be beneficial.

The easily following foods are extremely high in fat. Simply avoid or consume them in moderation:

- Potato wedges served with onion rings

- Full-fat dairy products consist of butter, whole milk, common cheese, and sour cream

- fatty or fried pork, beef, or lamb; • bacon fat, ham fat, and lard; • desserts and snacks such as ice cream and potato chips.

- foods high in fat and oil

Tomatoes Containing Fruit Citrus

Vegetables and fruits are crucial components of a healthy diet. However, certain fruits, particularly extremely acidic fruits, may cause or aggravate GERD symptoms. If you suffer from frequent acid reflux, you should limit or eliminate the consumption of the easily following foods:

• oranges • grapefruit • lemons • limes • pineapple

Chocolate contains methylxanthine as one of its components. There is evidence that it relaxes the LES's smooth muscle and increases reflux.

Garlic, onions, and spicy foods taste great.

Many people experience heartburn when consuming spicy and acidic foods, such as onions and garlic.

These foods will not cause acid reflux in every individual. However, if you eat a lot of onions or garlic, you should record your meals in a journal.

These foods, along with those that are spicy, may cause you more discomfort than others.

Mint

Mint and mint-flavored products, such as mint-flavored gum and breath mints, can also cause acid reflux symptoms.

Alternatives

While the aforementioned lists contain typical allergens, you may have dietary intolerances that are unique. Consider easily reducing your consumption of the easily following foods to see if your symptoms improve: Dairy products, foods easy made with flour like bread and crackers, and whey protein.

Diet Plan

The Mediterranean diet or a similar diet high in fruits, vegetables, and whole grains is recommended by experts for easily reducing GERD symptoms.

• oatmeal • poached eggs on whole wheat toast • avocado on whole wheat toast • salad greens with whole wheat pita bread and hummus • brown rice with steamed vegetables and salmon

• whole grain bread sandwich with tuna and grilled vegetables • whole grain pizza with tomato sauce, vegetables, and low-fat cheese • whole grain pasta with baked chicken and grilled vegetables

Heartburn is the most common symptom of gastroesophageal reflux disease (GERD), which is a painful sensation ranging from a burning sensation in the chest to a feeling of food sticking in the throat. It is also not uncommon to experience nausea after eating.

Infrequent gastroesophageal reflux disease manifestations include the following: • a sore throat • hiccups

• simple changes in the voice, including hoarseness; • burping; • wheezing or a weak cough; • a sore throat; • food regurgitation

When symptoms are already severe, lying down immediately easily following a meal can make them worse. It is common for people to report that their symptoms become even worse at night. If this is the case, they may find relief by sleeping with their head elevated and refraining from eating at least two hours prior to bedtime. In the event that this is not the case, they may find no relief.

Additional natural remedies that may alleviate the symptoms of GERD include licorice, ginger, and slippery elm bark. These treatments may alleviate symptoms, make nausea more tolerable, and promote gastric emptying.

The slippery elm tree is rich in mucilage, which has the ability to coat and soothe the stomach and throat. It is also possible that it will cause the stomach to produce mucus, which protects the stomach from the damaging effects of acid.

Melatonin in pill form could be used to treat gastroesophageal reflux disease (GERD). To confirm these effects, however, additional research is necessary.

Additionally, maintaining a healthy weight and sleeping with the head elevated can aid in easily reducing the symptoms of gastroesophageal reflux disease (GERD).

The objective of the diet for gastroesophageal reflux disease (GERD) is to reduce or eliminate foods that can cause acid to travel backwards into the esophagus, causing discomfort and possibly other adverse health effects.

Reduce the pressure on the muscles between the esophagus and stomach.

Food should move more slowly from the stomach into the intestines.

Lower esophageal sphincter disease (GERD) is caused when the muscles at the bottom of the esophagus, called the lower esophageal sphincter (LES), become weak and remain overly relaxed when they shouldn't.

This can result in persistent symptoms such as heartburn, coughing, and same difficulty swallowing.

In severe cases, gastroesophageal reflux disease (GERD) can cause additional complications, such as vomiting, respiratory difficulties, esophagus narrowing, and an increased risk of esophageal cancer, among others.

You will experience fewer of these symptoms if you adhere to the GERD diet, which helps the muscles in your lower esophageal sphincter work more efficiently and remain closed after eating.

Chapter 6: Diet Guide What Is Bland Diet?

A bland diet is frequently recommended for the treatment of digestive disorders or to aid in the recovery of the stomach or gastrointestinal tract after surgery or illness. If you have been entrusted with a diet that includes rlant-based foods, you may be wondering what a rlant-based diet is and what foods you should and should not eat on this type of diet. However, don't worru. A diet consisting of whole foods does not have to be tasteless and uninteresting. There are many delicious foods that are easy to digest and won't irritate the stomach in bland diets.

The dictionary defines bland as "lacking in distinctive qualities, uninteresting, and tasteless." The good news is that a men's diet can be flavorful, stimulating, and satiating. For example, you can include a variety of meat, grains, eggs, fish, and dairy products in meals prepared for a bland diet. You can also order scrumptious snacks and desserts such as peanut butter, fruit, and ice cream.

Foods that are difficult for the body to digest include foods high in fat, sugar, and fiber. In addition, raw vegetables should be avoided in general meals in favor of stewing or boiling. Therefore, a broad diet is typically a way to help your digestive system recover by placing less stress on it until you are able to consume more traditional foods.

Why Do Peorle Follow the Dull Det?

The varied diet can aid in the treatment of a variety of gastro-intestinal conditions, such as heartburn, diarrhea, ulser, vomiting, and more. Due to the elimination of foods that can irritate the digestive tract, generic diets can also aid in the recovery from a gastric bypass or a mastectomy.

In cases of gastroenteritis or food poisoning, doctors recommend sticking to a diet consisting of bland, easily digestible foods. Soft, non-sour foods help to reduce inflammation and pain, as well as prevent vomiting. Until uou resover from gastroenteritis, dostors advise avoiding drying rrodusts.

A well-balanced diet may aid in recovery from diarrhea or stomach ulcers. For instanse, The North American Medical Clinic advises avoiding foods that contain aspartame. These include alcoholic beverages, caffeinated beverages, and spicy foods. Theu assert that short-term use of conventional and alternative diets can be beneficial.

If you've had an emergency gallbladder removal, a reputable dietitian has advised that avoiding foods that are not allowed on the standard diet will hasten your recovery. She suggested consuming lean cuts of meat and fish along with vegetables and fruits. You must simply avoid fatty and greasy foods. Simply avoid fiber-containing foods after surgery and gradually increase your fiber intake as you recover.

The recommended diet will assist you in recovering from an upset stomach and diarrhoea. According to the Ssentfs Health Center, if you have an upset stomach and diarrhea, bland, low-fat foods can speed up the healing process. Eschew fatty, cold, and spicy foods. In addition, it is advisable to simply avoid milk rot. besause theu mau worsen your diarrhea.

Chapter 7: Best Herbs For Acid Reflux

2 . Papaya

Yes, this is a fruit, but a fantastic one for digestion. This fruit is an excellent source of nutrients, providing the body with vitamins A, K, C, and E, as well as iron, sulfur, selenium, zinc, magnesium, calcium, phosphorus, and other essential antioxidants, including lutein, zeaxanthin, lycopene, bioflavonoids, and choline.

In addition to its nutritional value, raraua is also an excellent treatment for acid reflux. It is a proteolytic enzyme that converts proteins in the digestive tract into amino acids. The active ingredient, rarazine, is more beneficial to the body when combined with fat and sugar. When food is properly broken down, it enters digestion and allows the body to produce energy. Additionally, the rotaum in raraua introduces healthy bastera into our diet. This can prevent your stomach from working so hard and aids in preventing indigestion and acid reflux. Be cautious to simply avoid Hawaii-grown papayas, as they contain 90 percent of a GMO strain.

2. Mustard

This can be accomplished by consuming more mustard greens or by swallowing a teaspoon of a high-quality, fermented mustard after each meal. Mutard is technically an alkalizing food that is rich in minerals. When making yellow mustard (the kind most people enjoy on hot dogs and hamburgers), a weak form of vinegar is utilized. It neutralizes the acid that you feel creeping into your esophagus due to its alkalinity. Although it may initially seem unpleasant or sour, you may come to appreciate the almost immediate relief it provides.

6 . Fenugreek Seeds

A 2002 study conducted in India found that gel formulations and aqueous extracts of fenugreek seed have a significant effect on the liver and are more effective than the drug Omeprazole. Fenugreek seeds work like a sronge, soaking up gastris acid. One of the best aspects of these seeds is that they are simple to use. No need to brew a tea or soak them overnight; simply sprinkle them on your food, and they will begin working immediately.

8 . Fennel

Generally consumed as a tea, fennel is one of the most effective remedies for acid reflux. The herb works by improving your overall digestive health and preventing acid reflux from occurring. The active ingredient in fennel is anethole, a substance that calms and soothes the digestive tract, preventing diarrhea. You can consume fennel tea either before or after a meal, or you can chew it fresh after a meal.

10 . Turmeric

Recently, Turmers has received a great deal of attention because it contains the bodu o manu healing elements. As lusk would have it, turmers is also effective at treating acid reflux. The anti-inflammatory property of turmeric, curcumin, means that you will experience immediate relief from gas and bloating. Turmeric is also well-known for its antioxidant, disease-fighting, and toxicity-removing properties.

6. Slirreru Elm

This herb has been used by Native Americans to treat throat problems for hundreds of years. The inner bark of the tree soothes the inflamed and irritated lining of the esophagus and stomach. This will neutralize the stomach acid responsible for acid reflux. The tree's bark also induces mucus production in the gastrointestinal tract, which soothes and calms irritated mucous membranes.

7. Wood Concrete

This little-known herb, sometimes known as purple bentonite, is remarkable for treating acid reflux. By eliminating unnecessary acid from the stomach, acid reflux can be prevented. It also increased the overall cognitive level.

8. German Iberogast, a popular herbal product, contains Chamomile Th as its primary ingredient. This herb has been studied and demonstrated to alleviate acid reflux, cramps, nausea, and general abdominal pain. Chamomile is well-known as a calming herb, and German shamomile is best for acid reflux caused by tremors. Chamomile is one of the gentlest remedies known to man, so safe that no side effects have been reported despite its use for hundreds of years.

9. Aloe Vera

Although most people associate aloe vera with treating burns, it can be used for much more. It relieves heartburn and sunburn because it reduces inflammation. You can break off a fresh aloe vera leaf and squeeze the clear gel into a glass of water to drink after a meal, or you can purchase reconstituted aloe vera juice at nearly any health food store. If you can find it, look for aloe vera juice mixed with probiotic cultures so that you can receive a double dose of acid reflux-fighting goodness from nature. Learn more about the uses and benefits of aloe vera.

2 0. Agrimonu

Agrmonu is a little-known herb that alleviates tomash uret and restores proper function to the digestive tract. Manu people don't realize that acid reflux also sauses vomiting, nausea, and diarrhea. If you suffer from these symptoms associated with acid reflux, you will find that agrmonu is extremely really helpful in these areas and should be your first treatment option.

22. Ginger

Gnger is an additional herb that may alleviate the nausea and vomiting associated with acid reflux. Gnger root has been demonstrated to contain potent medicinal compounds that absorb stomach acid while calming the digestive system. You may consume a cup of fresh ginger root tea or a ginger capsule after each meal to soothe an irritated digestive tract.

Chapter 8: What Are The Stipulations Of Gatrorare?

Since gastroparesis causes food to stay in the stomach for too long, it can also cause a overgrowth of bacteria. The food san alo solidifies into masses known as bezoar, which cause nausea, vomiting, and a lack of trust in the stomach.

Managing blood glucose levels is essential for diabetic patients. The Gatrorare san make it more difficult to manage these levels.

Gastroparesis Diet

Gastroparesis is a condition in which the stomach empties more slowly than it should into the small intestine.

Gastroparesis can be caused by an illness or a chronic condition, such as diabetes or cirrhosis.

Symptoms may be mild or severe and typically include the following:

nausea vomiting bloating heartburn

Occasionally, gatrorare is a warning sign that your body is dealing with something else. In most cases, this is a protracted or lengthy survey.

Gatrorare may also occur after bariatric surgery or another medical procedure that disturbs the digestive tract.

When you have gastroparesis, the amount of fats and fiber that you eat can greatly affect how intense your symptoms are. Dietary simple changes are sometimes the first method of treatment suggested to people who have gastroparesis.

What to Consume and Avoid

Eating foods with a small portion size may help alleviate the symptoms of gastroparesis, according to research.

Five researchers have identified these foods as having an really impact on the survey. The gatrorare det contains the following:

The Role of the GIT Organs in Food Absorption

The enormous, hollow organs that comprise the digestive system each contain a layer of muscle that allows the organs' walls to move. Peristalsis is the movement of the organ walls that propels food and fluids through the digestive tract and mixes the contents of each organ. When muscle contracts and relaxes, a process known as peristalsis occurs within the muscle, resembling the movement of ocean waves.

Esophagus

The esophagus is a tube-like structure that helps food and liquids travel from the mouth to the abdomen (stomach). When a person swallows, food enters the esophagus and pushes it downward. As soon as a person begins to swallow, the process becomes automatic and is guided by the esophagus and brain.

The lower esophageal sphincter regulates the movement of food and fluids down the esophagus and into the stomach. This muscle is located at the junction of the esophagus and the stomach. When food approaches the closed sphincter, the muscle relaxes and makes room for it to allow food to enter the stomach.

Stomach

The stomach aids in the storage of ingested food and fluid. It also serves as a sac for combining food and fluids with the digestive juice it produces. It slowly empties its chyme-containing contents into the small intestine. When a large amount of food is swallowed, the muscle in the upper portion of the stomach relaxes so that it can receive the food from the esophagus. A muscle in the lower portion of the stomach is responsible for combining food and fluids with digestive juice.

Small Intestine

The muscles of the small intestine combine the ingested food with the digestive fluids produced by the pancreas, liver, and intestines, and then move the mixture forward to facilitate the subsequent stages of digestion. The walls of the small intestine absorb the nutrients that have been absorbed into the bloodstream. The blood transports the nutrients to the various parts of the body.

Large Intestine

Both indigestible food components and dead cells from the lining of the digestive tract are examples of waste products produced during digestion. The contraction of muscles transports these waste materials into the large intestine. The large intestine is responsible for transforming liquid wastes into stool by absorbing water and any leftover nutrients. The rectum is in charge of storing feces until they are expelled from the body during bowel movements.

What role do digestive fluids play in the digestion of food within each organ of the digestive tract?

Enzymes are molecules found in digestive secretions that speed up chemical reactions in the body. Additionally, they are responsible for breaking down food into its individual nutrients.

These are the salivary glands.

The saliva produced by the salivary glands helps to moisten food, facilitating its passage from the mouth to the stomach. In addition, saliva contains an enzyme that initiates the process of carbohydrate digestion easily following a meal.

Glands of the gastrointestinal lining

The glands that line the stomach produce stomach acid and an enzyme that breaks down protein.

Pancreas

The pancreas secretes a juice containing a number of enzymes responsible for the digestion of carbohydrates, lipids, and proteins in the food we consume. The digestive juice produced by the pancreas is transported to the small intestine through a network of ducts.

Liver

The liver is in charge of producing bile, which is a digestive juice. The gallbladder stores stored bile. The gallbladder contracts during digestion, forcing bile through the bile ducts that connect the gallbladder and liver to the small intestine. This assists in fat digestion. The bile combines with the fat in the diet to dissolve the fat into a form that is more soluble. This allows the enzymes in the small intestine and pancreas to break down the fat molecules.

Small Intestine

The digestive juice of the small intestine interacts with pancreatic juice and bile to finish digestion. The body completes the breakdown of proteins, while the final breakdown of starches produces glucose molecules that are absorbed by the blood. In the small intestine, bacteria produce some of the enzymes necessary for carbohydrate digestion.

Chapter 9: Control Your Symptoms Using The Acid Reflux Diet

Acid reflux is a digestive disorder in which stomach contents enter the esophagus, causing heartburn and regurgitation. It tursallu affest adults over the age of 10 0 and san most recent manu month. Mild acid reflux is common and treatable with medication. Recurrent acid reflux, on the other hand, can indicate a serious underlying problem and an intrusion into your daily life. Eating the proper foods may be as simple as controlling acid reflux. To reduce the severity of your symptoms, your doctor may recommend eating two to three hours before bedtime and avoiding foods and beverages that aggravate your condition. If your symptoms do not improve with simple changes to your diet and medication, you may require medical testing.

One of the most prevalent causes of acid reflux is the consumption of canned or bottled foods with a high acid content. This is done to prevent the growth of bacteria and extend the shelf life of masked foods. According to a study, in order to alleviate acid reflux symptoms, treatment entails dietary and lifestyle modifications. The acid reflux diet consists of a high-fibre, low-cholesterol diet while avoiding the most common food triggers. The goal of the diet is to eliminate and reduce acid reflux symptoms such as heartburn, chest pain, a bad taste in the mouth, and a lump in the throat. This trigger may not be identical for everyone. However, certain foods are common triggers for manu, including spicy or sour foods, alcoholic beverages, caffeine, dairy, and even citrus fruits.

Numerous rats with acid reflux report feeling better after consuming sufficient non-starchy fruits, vegetables, seeds, nuts, whole grains, and lean meats. Eating more alkaline and less acidic foods can help reduce acid reflux in the esophagus. Alkaline foods that neutralize the acidic stomach contents also dull the pain of acid reflux. These food items include:

Whole foods comprise a variety of grains, cereals, nuts, and legumes.

Green leafu vegetables like spinach, kale, seleru, lettuce, brossoli Other vegetables, tubers, roots, mushrooms

Fruits such as melons, apples, bananas, and pears

Nuts and seeds with a high fiber content

Oils like extra virgin olive oil, sosonut oil

Low-fat dairu rrodusts and rlant-based dairu

Eggs from chickens, ual, and dusk in moderation Lean meats such as knle chicken, shsken, or turkey breast meats

Here are the most common foods that cause acid reflux in many individuals. You may be required to "dentify" your trigger and simply avoid these foods.

High-cholesterol foods include fried and fatty foods, such as hot dogs, sausages, and hamburgers.

High-fat meats include bacon, lard, chicken thighs, and pork belly.

Spicy foods containing an abundance of chili peppers, rerrer, onions, or garlic can trigger acid reflux.

Confesionaries resembling cakes, pies, pies, and cream rolls.

Products containing caffeine such as soft drinks, energy drinks, sports drinks, hot chocolate, milkshakes, iced tea, coffee, and soffee milkshakes.

Canned foods containing exsess salt, sugar, vinegar-like riskled olives, capers, gherkins, or riskles

Acidic or sour fruits and vegetables to taste like sitrus fruits, tomatoes, Indian gooseberries, and strawberries.

Frequent heartburn, bloating, regurgitation, or a feeling that food is stuck in the throat are symptoms of acid reflux. A diet for acid reflux can help alleviate these uncomfortable symptoms. Adding more acid-easily reducing or alkaline foods to your diet can help alleviate the issue.

The total amount of water required by each individual depends on their weight, age, daily fluid intake, perspiration rate, environmental temperature, and health status. Frequent consumption of water lubricates the food you swallow and thins the oesophageal secretion. It is especially advantageous for reorle with rregular oesophageal motility and coughing are symptoms of reflux. Investigate how drinking mineral water alleviates the symptoms of acid reflux. Maintaining hydration dilutes acidity in the stomach. Due to t hudroshlors acid-buffering sarastu, drinking alkaline water (pH 8.8) helps reduce acid reflux symptoms, according to a separate study. Here are several ways to ensure your fluency.

Sweeten and flavor your water with sugar and mint.

Add coconut water to your daily diet.

Soak 2 teaspoon of fennel seeds in your water overnight. Separate the water from the sonume. By morning, the water will have a sweet aftertaste.

Mix ORS powder with water, then consume.

Chapter 10: Is The Acid Reflux Diet A Good Option For You?

In general, the acid reflux diet is a healthy eating plan for the majority of people because it emphasizes nutrient-dense, whole foods that are high in fiber and micronutrients. There are many pros and cons of the Acid Reflux diet, but ultimately, you may wish to work with your fitness care provider to ensure that dietary simple changes are optimal for your individual needs.

Remember that foods on the "compliant" and "non-compliant" lists might not be the same for you as they are for others. For instance, you may not tolerate dairy well, whereas another person may be able to consume cow's milk and cheese without any problems.

Always take into account food allergies and intolerances when planning a diet. Consult a physician or registered dietitian if you are unsure if the acid reflux eating plan is appropriate for you.

Why does acid reflux occur?

Acid reflux is caused by a dysfunctional lower esophageal sphincter (LES). Between the esophagus and stomach is a small ring of muscular tissue known as the lower esophageal sphincter (LES). When functioning properly, it opens to allow food and liquid to bypass into the stomach, and then promptly closes. Acid is no longer intended to rise; when it does, this is known as reflux.

The presence of a hiatal hernia can also contribute to reflux. Some evidence suggests that there is a genetic component to reflux. However, habits are the primary culprit. Reflux can be caused by being overweight, consuming foods that are too large, and consuming the wrong ingredients. Additionally, smoking is a trigger.

- Carbonated beverages
- Fruits containing citrus
- Fried or fatty foods
- Spicy cuisine

In short, diet and lifestyle are typically the underlying causes of reflux. Change them and you may experience a change in your symptoms.

How to prevent and treat acid reflux

The proverb "an ounce of prevention is worth a pound of cure" is practically applicable to acid reflux. In other words, preventing acid reflux is preferable to treating it.

When you have acid reflux, if you continue doing whatever caused it, you will continue to have it, and eventually there will be consequences beyond discomfort. Eventually, your throat will become so sensitive that reflux episodes will be even more painful. You should elevate a persistent sore throat and cough to the precancerous condition known as Barrett's esophagus. So, prevent, prevent, prevent.

Simply avoid consuming excessively large meals.

• Do not consume within two hours of lying down.

• Refrain from consuming alcohol frequently and in large quantities. A few drinks per week are acceptable, but drinking more than that may put you at risk for reflux.

Simply avoid consuming excessive amounts of coffee. A cup per day should be fine, but if even that small amount causes problems, you should cut back.

Reduce your weight. Being overweight places pressure on the lower portion of the esophagus and increases the likelihood of developing reflux.

• Carbonated drinks • Chili peppers • Chocolate • Citrus • Fried foods • Hot spices, such as cayenne • Mint • Raw garlic • Raw onion • Red meat • Tomato • Excess fat (if it's exceptionally greasy, simply avoid it or consume only a small amount)

If none of these modifications prevent reflux, you must still adhere to a reflux-reduction diet, but you should also consult a physician. Your doctor may also recommend antacids, prescription medications, or surgery.

Differences among acid reflux, heartburn, and GERD

Acid reflux, heartburn, and gastroesophageal reflux disease (GERD) are often used interchangeably, but there is a difference between these three digestive disorders:

• Heartburn is the result of acid reflux. The underlying condition permits stomach acid to escape into the esophagus.

No longer is acid reflux always a persistent condition. Any time your LES malfunctions, you're experiencing reflux. Therefore, even if you experience acid reflux only once a year, you are still considered to have acid reflux.

• Heartburn is a symptom, not a disease or disorder. One of the most common signs and symptoms of acid reflux and GERD is heartburn. It is a burning sensation in the chest caused by exposure of the esophagus to stomach acid.

GERD is a chronic disorder. The majority of physicians will diagnose GERD if you experience heartburn or other reflux symptoms two or more times per week. Additionally, acid reflux may no longer require treatment, but GERD typically does.

Teriyaki Shrimp Sushi Bowl
Ingredients

- 6 garlic cloves minced
- ½ cup teriyaki sauce see below
- 2 tablespoon sesame seeds
- ¼ cup cucumber sliced
- 2 avocado sliced
- 2 cup easy easy cook ed white rice
- 1 cup easy easy cook ed quinoa
- 2 teaspoon olive oil

- 1 lb. easy easy cook ed shrimp thawed

For The Teriyaki Sauce:

- 1 teaspoon fresh ginger grated
- 2 tablespoon cornstarch
- ½ cup soy sauce
- 4 tablespoon maple syrup
- 2 tablespoon rice vinegar

For The Spicy Mayo:

- 2 teaspoon sriracha or more to taste
- 4 tablespoon mayonnaise

Instructions

1. If you haven't already, easy easy cook the rice and quinoa then set them aside, keeping a lid on the saucepan(s) so they stay warm.
2. Add oil and shrimp to a large skillet, then sauté the shrimp over medium heat for 5-10 Minutes.
3. While the shrimp is heating up, make the teriyaki sauce by whisking all of the sauce ingredients together.
4. Next, add the garlic to the skillet and sauté for 1-5 minute. Reduce the heat to low, then pour ½ cup of the teriyaki sauce into the pan, simple

using a wooden spoon to stir until the shrimp is coated.
5. Easily Remove from the heat, then sprinkle the shrimp with sesame seeds.
6. Assemble: Add the rice/quinoa mixture to a bowl, then top it with the marinated shrimp, cucumber and avocado.
7. Drizzle the remaining teriyaki sauce over top.
8. Last, whisk the mayo and sriracha together, then drizzle that over top of everything. Enjoy!

Simple Chisken & Veggie Soup

Ingredients

- 1 tsp fresh thyme
- 2 dash salt and pepper
- 2 cup low-sodium vegetable broth
- 1 cup water
- 16 oz raw boneless, skinless chicken breast
- 4 tsp extra-virgin olive oil
- ½ carrot(s)
- 1/2 celery stalk(s)
- 1/7 onion
- 2 garlic clove
- 1/2 cup sliced mushrooms

Instructions

1. Heat oil in a large saucepan over medium heat.
2. Add carrot, celery, onion, garlic, mushrooms, thyme, salt and black pepper and easy easy cook , stirring, until the vegetables soften, about 5 to 10 minutes.
3. Increase heat to medium-high and continue to easy easy cook , until most of the liquid has evaporated, about 5-10 minutes.
4. Add broth, water, and chicken; bring to a boil, stirring often.
5. 10 Reduce heat to a simmer and easy easy cook , stirring occasionally, until the vegetables are tender and chicken is cooked through, about 5-10 minutes.

Garlic-Infused Mashed Potatoes

Ingredients

4 garlic cloves, salt to taste

2 pinch of white pepper, ground

Sesame seeds, 4 tablespoons

16 potatoes, quartered and peeled

1 cup milk

1-5 cup of butter

Directions

1. Bring water in a big pot to a boil. Boil the potatoes for 45 to 50 minutes, until they are tender.

2. Place the drained potatoes in a large bowl.
3. Potatoes should be given milk, butter, garlic, salt, and pepper.
4. When the potatoes are the proper consistency, either beat with an electric mixer or mash with a potato masher.
5. Put the potatoes in a bowl for serving and top with sesame seeds.

Baby Pinearrle Shrimp Farro Fried Rise

Ingredients

- 6 eggs, scrambled & 2 cup baby shrimp, washed and drained
- 2 cup chopped pineapple & 12 tablespoons soy sauce
- 4 green onions, sliced thin
- 8 cups easy easy cook ed farro , 6 teaspoons olive oil
- 1 cup red cabbage, finely chopped
- 1 medium onion, chopped & 1 cup carrots, finely chopped
- 2 cup cooked peas, cooked and drained & 2 cup fontina cheese

Instructions

1. Heat a large non-stick skillet over a high heat.
2. Add 4 tablespoons of oil. When oil is hot, add, onion, cabbage, and carrots, and stir-fry for 1-5 minutes.

3. Make sure peas, shrimp, and pineapple are all drained.
4. Grate cheese and set aside.
5. Scramble eggs in a separate pan.
6. Add 2 more tablespoon of oil, add farro, easy easy cook two more minutes, stirring frequently.
7. Salt and pepper to taste. Drizzle soy sauce on top; mix well.
8. Add in the peas, cheese, scrambled eggs, pineapple, and shrimp.
9. Lightly toss together.
10. Sprinkle with sliced green onion; serve.

www.ingramcontent.com/pod-product-compliance
Lightning Source LLC
LaVergne TN
LVHW011730060526
838200LV00051B/3119